Strength in Every Move

Resistant Band Workout for Women

Dr. Monica Haman

OTHER BOOKS BY THIS AUTHOR

https://www.amazon.com/dp/B0BRDGMMRB

https://www.amazon.com/dp/B0BSTMZ7PJ

https://www.amazon.com/dp/B0BT9912YX

https://www.amazon.com/dp/B0BRX25GC6

https://www.amazon.com/dp/B0BX2FRN1Q

TABLE OF CONTENTS

INTRODUCTION

Please accept my warm welcome to enter the world of "Strength in Every Move: Resistance Band Workout for Women." Because I'm a woman in my fifties who has dealt with self-doubt and body image issues, I know all too well the many problems that life brings us. This book is more than a set of exercises; it's a safe space created with compassion and understanding for ladies like you and me.

I can see you. I know that you have busy lives that don't leave much time for the gym, that you feel self-conscious in public places where you work out, and that physical problems like pregnancy, postpartum changes, and joint pain can seem impossible to get past. This book is for the fighter who wants to be healthier and stronger but is trying to keep up with the complicated dance of life.

In these pages, you'll find a safe place for women at all stages of their lives. These resistance band workouts can help you gain confidence and strength, whether you're starting the exciting journey of pregnancy, getting stronger again after giving birth, or just trying to get away from joint pain.

For active people looking for a new, exciting task, this book is your inspiration. It takes you away from the everyday and into the extraordinary. It's what I've been doing all my life, what I love, and what I believe in the power that we all have.

This is more than just an exercise guide; it's a friend, a confidante, and a constant source of support. It includes workouts for people of all fitness levels, from those who are just starting to get fit to those who are looking for a new challenge. We're celebrating the amazing strength that's inside us, just waiting to be let out.

It's for us, the fighters, the moms, the thinkers, and the seekers. Let's find power in every move and love our bodies, stories, and what it means to be a woman. You've arrived in a world where working out is more than just a habit; it's a party. Let's go on this trip together, and let each stretch, pull, and win remind us of how powerful we are.

We shall overcome.

Chapter One

Getting Started

Let's start a fitness journey together that will change the way you work out and how you feel about your body. We're going to lay the groundwork and learn more about resistance bands in this chapter. These simple but incredibly useful tools have changed my fitness routine and the fitness routines of many others.

Understanding the Basics: What Are Resistance Bands?

So, exactly what are resistance bands? Consider them your own personal gym. These bands, which are frequently constructed of rubber or latex, come in a variety of resistance levels. They're more than simply elastic strips; they're your ticket to a leaner, healthier self. There is a band for every fitness level, from gentle to strenuous.

Choosing the Right Band for You

It's important to pick the right band. Getting the right pair of shoes is like that; they have to fit just right. For starters, smaller resistance bands might be a good choice. As they get stronger, they can move on to heavier bands. The point is to push yourself without overworking your muscles hurt.

The Benefits of Resistance Bands: Why Choose Them?

Why should you use resistance bands? For starters, they are gentler on your joints than hefty weights, lowering your risk of injury. Furthermore, they engage many muscle groups at the same time, providing a thorough workout. Consider sculpting your arms, legs, and core with a single, simple band.

Incorporating Bands Into Your Routine: Making It Seamless

The adaptability of resistance bands is one of their best features. They can transform any room into your personal gym. We'll look at how to incorporate them into your regular routine, from morning stretches to focused muscle workouts. Convenience meets efficacy.

Preparing Your Mind and Body: Setting Realistic Goals

Finally, let us discuss goal setting. Having a specific exercise goal will keep you motivated. Having a goal in mind will motivate your determination, whether it's gaining strength, improving flexibility, or simply feeling healthier.

I'm delighted to accompany you through this phase. By the conclusion, you'll not only comprehend the power of resistance bands, but you'll also be ready to confidently begin your fitness adventure.

Chapter Two

Essential Exercises

This chapter will walk you through the steps of performing fundamental resistance band exercises that target specific muscle areas such as the ankles, hips, back, and shoulders. These exercises are intended to give a full-body workout that improves strength, stability, and flexibility.

Complete Body Warm-Up

Dynamic stretching:

1. To loosen up the muscles in your upper body, start with arm swings, shoulder rolls, and neck rotations.

2. To activate the core, go to side bends, waist twists, and trunk rotations.

3. To warm up the muscles in your lower body, use leg swings, knee lifts, and ankle rolls.

Resistance Band Movements

1. Put the resistance band beneath each foot.

2. To warm up your arms and shoulders, try some light resistance band pulls.

3. To exercise your glutes and engage your hips, take side steps with the band.

Targeted Workouts: Arms, Core, Legs, Ankles, Hips, Back, and Shoulders

Arms: Bicep Curls

1. With your feet shoulder-width apart and the band handles in each hand, take a posture on the resistance band.

2. Curl the band upward while keeping your elbows close to your torso to flex your biceps.

3. Slowly lower the band while fully extending your arms. To the desired extent, repeat.

Tricep Extensions

1. With one foot planted on the resistance band and one hand held behind your head, take a stand.

2. Raise your arm and make sure it is completely straight.

3. Lower your hand behind your head slowly while maintaining a straight upper arm. After the required number of repetitions, swap sides and repeat.

Hammer Curls

1. Using both feet, stand on the resistance band and grasp a handle in each hand with the palms facing your thighs.

2. Curl the bands while keeping your upper arms still and clenching your biceps.

3. Return the bands to their starting positions slowly. To the desired extent, repeat.

Tricep Kickbacks

1. Stand on the resistance band with both feet, holding a handle in each hand, arms bent at 90 degrees.

2. Straighten your arms behind you, engaging your triceps.

3. Slowly return to the starting position. To the desired extent, repeat.

Core: Russian Twists

1. With your legs outstretched and both hands on the handles of the band, take a seat on the floor.

2. Using your core muscles, slant your head back a little.

3. With each twist, turn your torso to the right and then the left, making contact with the floor next to your hip. To the desired extent, repeat.

Plank with Resistance Band Row

1. With the resistance band looped around both wrists, take on the plank position.

2. Pull one hand toward your hip while keeping the plank position, using your back muscles.

3. Put the hand back in the plank position and switch sides. Keep your core steady throughout the exercise.

Bicycle Crunches with Resistance Band

1. While keeping your hands on the handles, loop the resistance band around your feet while lying on your back.

2. Raise your shoulders, feet, and head off the floor.

3. Switch sides in a pedaling action, alternating between moving your right elbow closer your left knee and straightening your right leg. Throughout the exercise, pay close attention to using your core muscles.

Resistance Band Woodchoppers

1. Secure the resistance band over your head at a fixed location.

2. Maintain a shoulder-width distance between your feet while grasping the band with both hands.

3. To work your obliques, twist your torso and drag the band diagonally across your body.

4. Get back to where you were before. For the required number of repetitions, repeat on both sides.

Legs: Resistance Band Squats

1. Holding the handles at shoulder height, place the resistance band beneath both feet.

2. Maintaining a straight back and raised chest, lower yourself into a squat position.

3. Engage your glutes and quadriceps as you push through your heels to stand back up. To the desired extent, repeat.

Resistance Band Leg Press

1. Attach the resistance band to a stable object on the ground.

2. Wrap the band around your feet while lying on your back.

3. Engage your quadriceps as you push your legs straight against the resistance. Return your knees to their initial position slowly. To the desired extent, repeat.

Resistance Band Side Steps

1. Encircle your ankles with the resistance band.

2. Put yourself in a semi-squat and bend your knees slightly.

3. Maintaining the band's tension as you take tiny side steps will help you engage your outer thighs and hips.

4. Take different routes. To the desired extent, repeat.

Resistance Band Step-Ups

1. Hold the grips at your sides and plant one foot in the middle of the resistance band.

2. With the banded foot, step onto a bench or other stable surface, fully straightening your leg.

3. Return the foot with the band to the ground. After the specified number of repetitions, switch sides and repeat.

Ankles: Resistance Band Ankle Flexion

1. With one leg extended and the other bowed, take a seat on the floor.

2. Wrap the resistance band around your foot's ball.

3. Extend your ankle and push against resistance to bring the band closer to you. Take a quick hold, then let go. After the required number of repetitions, swap sides and repeat.

Resistance Band Dorsiflexion

1. Stretching your legs out in front of you, wrap the resistance band first around your foot and then around a stationary point.

2. To flex your ankle, pull your toes towards you against the resistance.

3. Take a quick hold, then let go. After the specified number of repetitions, switch sides and repeat.

Resistance Band Eversion and Inversion

1. Stretching your legs out, take a seat on the floor.

2. Encircle one of your ankles and a stationary point with the resistance band.

3. Eversion is rotating your foot outward against resistance; inversion is rotating it inward.

4. Take a quick hold, then let go. After the specified number of repetitions, switch sides and repeat.

Resistance Band Plantarflexion

1. Stretch your legs apart while sitting on the floor, then wrap the resistance band over one foot's ball.

2. Toe-pointing, press your foot down against the resistance.

3. Take a quick hold, then let go. After the specified number of repetitions, switch sides and repeat.

Hips: Resistance Band Hip Abduction

1. Encircle your ankles with the resistance band.

2. Maintaining tension in the band, place your feet hip-width apart.

3. Using your hip muscles, raise one leg sideways against the resistance. Quickly hold and let go. 4. 4.

4. After the required number of repetitions, swap sides and repeat.

Resistance Band Glute Kickbacks

1. With the resistance band looped around one foot, get on your hands and knees.

2. Kick your leg backward against resistance while maintaining a 90-degree bend in your knee and using your glutes.

3. Return your leg to its initial position by lowering it. After the specified number of repetitions, switch sides and repeat.

Resistance Band Hip Flexion

1. Wrap the resistance band around your ankles while lying on your back.

2. Maintaining your legs straight, raise them off the ground.

3. In order to overcome the resistance, flex your hips and bring your knees close to your chest. Lower your legs again after a few moment of holding. To the desired extent, repeat.

Resistance Band Hip Thrusts

1. With a resistance band coiled slightly above your knees and your upper back resting against a bench, take a seat on the floor.

2. Plant your feet firmly on the ground and bend your knees.

3. Lift your hips towards the sky by pushing through your heels and push your knees outward against the resistance.

4. Reposition your hips lower. To the desired extent, repeat.

Back: Resistance Band Rows

1. At chest height, secure the resistance band around a robust object.

2. With both hands on the band handles, face the anchor point.

3. In order to squeeze your shoulder blades together, pull the bands towards your chest. Once you've completed the required number of repetitions, slowly let go.

Resistance Band Lat Pulldowns

1. Underneath the resistance band, sit or kneel, and secure it overhead.

2. With both hands, hold the band while extending your arms upward.

3. Engage your upper back and lats muscles as you pull the band down towards your chest. Repeat after releasing slowly.

Resistance Band Face Pulls

1. Wrap the resistance band around a stationary object that is at chest height.

2. With your arms extended forward, grasp the band handles in each hand.

3. While maintaining your upper arms parallel to the floor, pull the bands towards your face. Repeat by slowly releasing and then squeezing your shoulder blades together again.

Resistance Band Deadlifts

1. Grasping a handle in each hand, take a stand with both feet on the resistance band.

2. Lower your torso by bending at the hips and knees, maintaining a flat back.

3. Pull the bands towards your thighs as you straighten your hips and knees and stand back up.

4. After you've completed the required number of repetitions, gradually reduce the bands.

Shoulders: Resistance Band Shoulder Press

1. Holding the handles at shoulder height, take a stand on the resistance band.

2. As you fully stretch your arms overhead, push the bands upward.

3. Reposition the bands so they are shoulder height. To the desired extent, repeat.

Resistance Band Lateral Raises

1. Grasp the handles at your sides while standing with both feet on the resistance band.

2. Raise your arms straight to shoulder height while contracting your lateral deltoids.

3. Relative to your sides, lower your arms. To the desired extent, repeat.

Resistance Band Shoulder External Rotation

1. With both feet planted firmly on the resistance band, place your hand by your side and grasp one end.

2. Rotate your forearm outward, away from your body, against the resistance, while maintaining your elbow near to your body.

3. Return to the starting position slowly. After the specified number of repetitions, switch sides and repeat.

Resistance Band Front Raises

1. Using both feet, stand on the resistance band and grasp the handles with your palms facing your thighs.

2. Raise the bands to shoulder height right in front of you while maintaining a straight arm position.

3. Bring the bands down to your thighs again. To the desired extent, repeat.

Remember to keep perfect form, move with control, and adjust the resistance of the band to your fitness level. A resistance band workout that incorporates a variety of exercises offers a well-rounded and effective workout.

Chapter Three

Advanced Workouts

In this chapter, we'll explore the thrilling world of advanced resistance band workouts, a place where your willpower meets the challenge and transformation awaits. Advanced workouts are more than just physical challenges; they are transformative experiences that shape your strength, endurance, and mental fortitude. As I offer these activities, I want you to know that I've been there. I've felt the burn, the tiredness, and the tremendous exhilaration that comes from pushing my own boundaries. Allow me to guide you not only as a doctor, but also as someone who has sweated, faltered, and succeeded alongside you.

Cardio with Bands

Consider your heartbeat synchronising with the rhythm of your motions. Cardio with resistance bands accomplishes this. I could hardly do a minute of jumping jacks with bands when I first started. But with perseverance, I discovered that my stamina was increasing. I progressed from simple movements to sophisticated, heart-pounding sequences.

Resistance band jumping jacks, squat leaps, and lateral shuffles, for example, not only improve your cardiovascular fitness but also challenge your coordination. Don't be disheartened if you find yourself short of breath at first. Remember that with each pant, your body adapts, grows stronger, and becomes more efficient.

High-Intensity Workouts

High-intensity workouts may appear intimidating, yet they are extremely empowering. Consider doing resistance band burpees or mountain climbers. These workouts, while strenuous, are quite effective. I struggled at first to keep up, but I didn't give up. I persevered, and you will as well. The burning sensation is caused by your muscles evolving and your body becoming more resilient.

As your endurance improves, you'll find yourself lasting longer, pushing harder, and feeling less tired. The sense of success that comes from completing a high-intensity workout is unrivalled. It's a celebration of your mental fortitude as much as your physical power.

Each drop of sweat, each increased heartbeat, is a brush stroke that shapes your endurance and strength. Don't compare your first chapter to someone else's tenth. Accept your path, enjoy your accomplishments, and don't be discouraged by brief setbacks. Even if you are tired, showing up and doing what you can is an accomplishment in and of itself.

Also keep in mind that stamina does not increase overnight. It's a steady process, with minor successes along the way. Don't get disheartened by the early difficulties. Accept the discomfort as a sign that you're pushing yourself. Those moments of struggle can be transformed into moments of triumph with constant effort. The ability to hold a plank for a few seconds longer, or to perform an extra set of jumping jacks, are examples of progress. Commemorate them.

So, as you venture into the area of advanced workouts, keep in mind that you are capable of far more than you believe. With each resistance band-assisted push-up, squat, and high knee, you're growing mental fortitude as well as physical strength. You're growing stronger, more determined, and unstoppable.

Chapter Four

Special Cases

This chapter explores the distinct landscapes of pregnancy, postpartum recovery, and joint health. Life's ups and downs frequently necessitate specialised care, and I've written this piece with profound understanding and compassion.

Exercises for Pregnancy and Postpartum:

Pregnancy: Carrying life within you is nothing short of amazing. Consider including activities that not only preserve your strength but also strengthen your relationship with your growing kid during these wonderful months.

Begin your practise with relaxing pregnant yoga practises, breathing deeply to surround your baby in peace. Switch to seated resistance band workouts to not only tone your arms but also to remind yourself of your persistent power. As you improve, embrace the healing potential of pelvic tilts to relieve the strain on your lower back. Practise this exercise three times per week, allowing these moments of conscious movement to serve as a refuge for you and your unborn child.

Postpartum: Exercises that gently guide you back into your body, promoting resilience and self-assurance, are required during the postpartum time, a chapter of soft healing and rediscovery.

Begin your practise by breathing diaphragmatically, centering yourself in the rhythm of inhales and exhales and connected with your core. Progress into resistance band squats as a declaration of your renewed strength, which is necessary for bearing both your baby and the world. Accept the transformational power of pelvic floor exercises combined with resistance band arm lifts to affirm the beauty of your changing body. Devote 20 minutes four times a week to this self-love practise, acknowledging each action as a step towards rekindling your confidence and vitality.

Tailored Workouts for Joint Health

Arthritis Relief: These activities provide solace and gentle fortitude to those suffering from arthritis pain. Begin with sitting leg lifts, a subtle compliment to your lower limbs' strength. Move into seated resistance band rows as a physical act, but also as a testimonial to your inner strength. Finish with seated knee extensions, breathing through the stretches and gently coaxing your joints into flexibility. Embrace these exercises on a daily basis, taking 15 minutes to honour your body's inherent knowledge and elegance.

General Joint Health: Maintaining joint mobility necessitates a multifaceted technique that combines strength and suppleness.

Begin your ritual with five minutes of gentle cardio, synchronising your heartbeat with the rhythm of your body's energy. Transition into resistance band shoulder rotations, which are an ode to your upper body's suppleness. Progress to standing hip abductions, each lift highlighting your hips' natural power. Finish with ankle circles as a gentle nod to your foundation. Dedicate 15 minutes to this routine three times a week as a significant expression of your dedication to your body's long-term wellness.

These exercises are about more than simply physical motions; they are also about self-discovery and acceptance. These exercises are woven with care, whether you're nourishing life within you, regaining your body after the glorious turmoil of childbirth, or tending to the precise requirements of your joints. They are an invitation to go deeper into yourself, to embrace your flaws, and to appreciate your strength.

Through this book, I offer you my unwavering empathy and support.

Chapter Five

Nutrition and Recovery

As we delve deeper into the world of resistance band workouts, it's critical to address an issue that is frequently overlooked: nutrition and recovery. Our bodies are amazing engines that require the necessary fuel to work optimally as well as the proper care to recover after exercise. In this chapter, I'll share insights not only as the author, but also as someone who has firsthand experience with the transforming impacts of mindful diet and recovery.

Eating Right for Your Workouts

Consider your body to be a garden. It need the proper nutrition to thrive, including a well-balanced diet of proteins, carbs, healthy fats, vitamins, and minerals. Consider a light snack high in carbohydrates and protein before your activity.

This mixture fuels your muscles and gives you long-lasting energy. After your workout, consume a post-exercise meal rich in lean meats, whole grains, and veggies. Consider it like nurturing your plant after a bright day - it aids in muscle regeneration and growth.

Hydration is also essential. Water is more than just a beverage; it is liquid vitality. Continue to sip throughout the day, especially during workouts. Dehydration can deplete your energy and slow your development. Additionally, during strenuous activities, consider consuming electrolyte-rich liquids to replace minerals lost through sweat.

Recovery Tips After Exercising

Let us now discuss recuperation. It is not just about resting; it is also about active renewal. Stretching after a workout is similar to gardening in that it develops flexibility and prevents discomfort. Concentrate on the muscle areas you've worked, gradually inviting them to relax.

Dear readers, sleep is your body's nightly healing ritual. Aim for 7-9 hours of uninterrupted sleep. Your body repairs muscles and consolidates memories as you sleep, ensuring you wake up refreshed and ready to face the day's challenges.

Consider massage and foam rolling, which are similar to spa treatments for your garden. They improve blood flow, relax muscles, and aid in healing. Don't underestimate the healing potential of a warm bath loaded with Epsom salts; it's a soothing soak that relaxes both the body and the mind.

Finally, pay attention to your body's whispers. Give it rest if it craves it. If it requests for food, give it nutritious food. Your body understands what it need; all we need to do is learn its language.

In essence, nurturing your body is as important as exercising. A well-fed and well-rested body, like a flourishing garden, blossoms with vigour, resilience, and enduring beauty. So, my dear readers, let us not just exercise; let us nurture not just our muscles, but our entire being.

Chapter Six

Staying Motivated

In this chapter, we'll look at the driving force behind any fitness journey: motivation. As someone who has personally experienced the transformational impact of hip resistance bands, I am well aware of the ups and downs that come with the territory. It's not just about the physical exertion; it's also about the mental and emotional journey towards a healthier, stronger you.

Setting Goals

Setting specific, attainable goals is identical to charting a course on a map. It provides your fitness journey meaning and direction. Resistance band training goals might range from toning specific muscle regions to improving endurance or simply feeling more active in your daily life.

Begin with simple, attainable goals that are in line with your ambitions. perform you want to perform 10 more squats? Do you want to learn a difficult resistance band move? Setting these goals, no matter how insignificant they may appear, can provide a sense of accomplishment, motivating you ahead.

However, objectives are about more than simply the destination; they are also about the journey. Celebrate your wins, no matter how tiny they appear to be. Each extra rep, each session completed, is a victory worth celebrating. These minor victories are the stepping stones to your larger aspirations.

Overcoming Challenges

Challenges, oh challenges, the stepping stones to resilience. We all face obstacles, whether they are time limits, a lack of enthusiasm, or unforeseen occurrences. The trick is not to escape these difficulties, but to face them with grace and commitment.

When your motivation wanes, remember why you started this trip in the first place. Consider the version of yourself you want to be. Perhaps it's the strong, confident woman effortlessly completing her workouts, or the vivacious soul eager to enjoy life's adventures. Keep that image in mind. In times of doubt, use it as a lighthouse.

Surround yourself with positive people. Whether it's a helpful friend, a motivating fitness community, or even a motivational quotation, these sources of optimism can rekindle your determination when it's on the verge of fading.

Remember, my reader, that every stumble is an opportunity to stand taller. Every obstacle is an opportunity to get stronger. Resistance band workouts are about more than simply physical transformation; they are about uncovering the depths of your own power, perseverance, and resolve. Never forget the incredible trip you're on as you face the challenges. You're shaping your spirit as well as your body, one resistance band at a time.

Chapter Seven

Sample Workouts

Welcome to a chapter that focuses on the practical aspects of our resistance band adventure. Now that we've covered the fundamentals and improved our skills, it's time to put our knowledge to use with these expertly created sample exercises.

These workouts are more than just exercises; they are the sum of our knowledge, focused at moulding your body and increasing your fitness levels. These workouts were created with progression in mind, catering to a variety of fitness levels and goals. So, grab your resistance bands and join me on a revolutionary fitness adventure.

Beginner's Full-Body Routine

This introductory workout will introduce you to the world of resistance band workouts. It's designed for beginners, with an emphasis on laying a solid foundation and maintaining appropriate form. Let's start by engaging our muscles with a thorough warm-up to ensure our bodies are prepared for the trials ahead.

1. Warm-Up (5 minutes):

    Jumping jacks to elevate heart rate.

    Arm circles and wrist rotations to warm up upper body.

    Bodyweight squats and lunges to engage lower body.

2. Resistance Band Exercises (20 minutes):

- Bicep Curls: 3 sets of 12 repetitions.

- Squats with Band: 3 sets of 15 repetitions.

- Seated Rows: 3 sets of 12 repetitions.

- Plank with Band Row: 3 sets of 10 repetitions per arm.

3. Cool Down and Stretching (5 minutes):

- Neck, shoulder, and arm stretches.

- Seated hamstring stretch and quadriceps stretch.

- Deep breathing exercises for relaxation.

Intermediate Strength Building

After you've mastered the fundamentals, this intermediate workout focuses on increasing strength and endurance. We'll increase the intensity of the exercises while emphasising controlled movements and proper posture.

1. Warm-Up (5 minutes):

   - Jumping jacks, mountain climbers, and dynamic lunges.

   - Shoulder rolls and wrist flexors to prepare the upper body.

2. Resistance Band Exercises (25 minutes):

   - Tricep Kickbacks: 3 sets of 12 repetitions per arm.

- Resistance Band Push-Ups: 3 sets of
  10 repetitions.

- Lateral Raises: 3 sets of 15
  repetitions.

- Resistance Band Squats with
  Overhead Press: 3 sets of 12
  repetitions.

3. Cool Down and Stretching (5 minutes):

   - Spinal twists, hip flexor stretch, and
     calf stretches.

   - Deep breathing and mindfulness
     exercises for mental relaxation.

Advanced Cardio and Endurance

This advanced workout incorporates cardiac aspects
and high-intensity activities, boosting your heart

rate and pushing your limits for those looking for a challenge.

1. Warm-Up (10 minutes):

   - Jumping jacks, high knees, and burpees for cardio activation.

   - Arm circles, wrist stretches, and ankle rotations for mobility.

2. Resistance Band Exercises (30 minutes):

   - Resistance Band Jump Squats: 4 sets of 15 repetitions.

   - High-Intensity Band Sprints: 3 sets of 30 seconds.

   - Mountain Climbers with Band Resistance: 3 sets of 20 repetitions.

   - Resistance Band Burpees: 3 sets of 12 repetitions.

3. Cool Down and Stretching (10 minutes):

   Full-body stretching focusing on major muscle groups.

   Yoga-inspired stretches for flexibility and relaxation.

   Deep breathing exercises for mental and physical recovery.

Remember that consistency is essential for growth. Pay attention to your body, remain hydrated, and nourish yourself properly. These sample workouts are more than just routines; they are landmarks in your fitness journey. Accept the trials, rejoice in the wins, and keep moving forward. Your greatest advantages are your strength and resilience. Have fun working out!